Versatile Role of Carcinosin

Key to its Uses

Nitesh Jain, M.D.
Former Asst. Prof. M.N.H. Medical College and Research Institute, Bikaner.

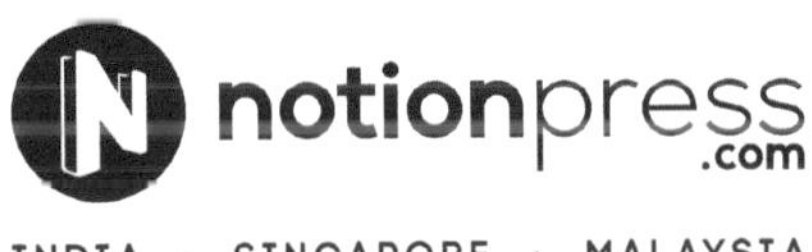

Notion Press Media Pvt Ltd

No. 50, Chettiyar Agaram Main Road,
Vanagaram, Chennai, Tamil Nadu - 600 095

First Published by Notion Press 2021

ISBN 978-1-63904-628-7

INITIAL REMARKS

During my initial days of Homoeopathic study I was perplexed to witness prescription of Carcinosin by some physicians simply to relieve the pain of carcinoma or to use it when they find the ancestral history or personal history of carcinoma; leaving aside the symptom totality. Although, much proving is conducted on Carcinosin still many Homoeopath are unable to take its full advantage that they could have taken, due to the seemingly antagonistic symptoms like – the person is too intelligent but can be mentally retarded, or he is mild and gentle or he is too much irritable and angry, creating much confusion in perceiving the real essence of the medicine and using it therapeutically. Thereby, I began to collect notes from various sources and use it in my practice and saw that like any other medicine Carcinosin can be given purely basing on its totality. Carcinosin has many symptoms that matches exactly with the well known polycrests, so whenever the case requires Carcinosin; many times other polycrest are employed and the case is approached in zigzag manner.

Gradually, practice showed that Carcinosin has versatile role to play, if used judiciously. It is so important medicine to use in today's modern lifestyle diseases that it cannot be kept aside. Those using it, will vouch for its efficiency. This book is result of my experiences with Carcinosin in variety of cases. Using this drug has always given me immense hope and confidence in what I perceive, hope "you too" add it in your armamentarium against diseases for benefit of mankind.

To start with this book begins with the portrait of Carcinosin followed by cases in which rubrics are mentioned in bracket depicting role of Carcinosin in Homeopathic therapeutics like it can be used –

- ❖ In carcinoma cases.
- ❖ In acute cases.
- ❖ In cases having direct cause effect relationship correlating to Carcinosin.
- ❖ In chronic jumbled up cases where indicated medicine does not act as expected.
- ❖ In those cases where well indicated medicine fails due to presence of some obstacle.
- ❖ In cases where constitutional indication of Carcinosin were seen.
- ❖ In cases where numerous polycrest medicines seems indicated.

In later part, the book has some serendipity of clinical symptoms by grace of almighty and my mentor Dr. (Prof) Himanshu Shekhar Rath who trained me to observe and major symptoms that I consider in prescribing

Carcinosin. In cases Placebo is also mentioned by Rubrum or Nihilinum, their doses depends on the circumstances.

Codes of references used in this work are –

- Complete repertory by Roger van Zandvoort – CR.
- Medical repertory by Robin Murphy – M.
- Aphorism from 6th edition of Organon of Medicine is shown by § sign.
- Organon Revisited by Nitesh Jain.

This book saw light due to inspiration of my senior Dr. Shivangi Jain, who constantly pushed me to write something, and Dr. Lakshmikanth Ponnuru, who managed his busy schedule and went through the manuscript. I am thankful to all the patients who kept their faith in me and Homoeopathy and shared even the most intimate things, due to which I could perceive more clearly.

Final thanks goes to my publisher Notion Press and Nikitha Lalwani, Yeshwini Doshi, Urmi Mukherjee for publishing this work in its present form, hope profession would gain much from it and help the ailing humanity.

Jai Homoeopathy.

Jai Bharat.

Nitesh Jain.

drniteshhomoeopath@gmail.com

CONTENTS

1. PORTRAIT OF CARCINOSIN

Older books says that in case of family history of carcinoma we can use Carcinosin, but in today's era there is hardly any family who will not be having family history of carcinoma so it cannot be taken up literally but if many persons in family have been suffering from carcinoma or they died of carcinoma at very young age, then Carcinosin should be thought of. Also, if there is family history of other genetic diseases, autoimmune diseases, DM, or Koch.

Modern world and its lifestyle have taken numerous people on earth in its grip leading to what we call lifestyle diseases. This medicine when used judiciously in today's scenario is the answer to many problems. We commonly hear that during pregnancy the lady is weak, suffers from hyperemesis gravidarum, anorexia or previously have had abortion or MTP due to varied reasons. Now when she again becomes pregnant; what would be her mental and physical condition! She will be in constant stress and anxieties that may the previous condition do not occur. These constant brooding over, leads to many problems in baby; at times amounting to congenital deformity or genetic diseases. Many cases of developmental delay have such history which needs to be taken care of. Some unmanageable problems during labour takes place and LSCS is done to save baby or mother from life threatening complications and baby is born prematurely. This premature baby is immunologically so weak that he could hardly survive in today world without support of his mother, so; he is kept in incubator away from his mother. This keeping of child in incubator away from mother puts an impact on his mental and physical being and he becomes vulnerable. This baby born in hospital suffers from neonatal jaundice and pneumonia, if not treated well pneumonia gets severe and reaches to dyspnoea, followed by asthma. Numerous such cases of premature birth is seen to have been suffering from Allergic rhinitis and they catch cold easily, since birth. Even if they eat ice cream or drink water soon after playing when drenched in sweat they suffer from sore throat and B/L tonsillitis. A premature born baby of 45 days was so sensitive that whenever her mother drank chilled drinks he gets fever and becomes completely sleepless (CR – Sleep, Sleeplessness, General Children, in) and kept on crying day in and day out. Carcinosin given to her mother taking her history cured this baby. (Hahnemann in Chronic diseases says that when baby is only on mother's milk then medicine should be given to mother.)

Children also become vulnerable due to their hard time in family if his father or mother, even grandparent is somewhat like "Hitler", always dominating and punishing (CR – Mentals, Ailments from domination from others, a long history of.). They are generally under extreme pressure created by their guardians to achieve what they could not achieve so they give them almost everything that is needed but not love and appreciation that they demand. They crave love and usually help others with an intention of receiving love in return, but when the expected love is not reciprocated their whole life becomes chaotic. This is generally seen in adolescent romantic love failure, when a breakup makes everything upside down. They then start to love pet animals and nature. Single child of family having his pet as best friend, always goes out with him and talks with him in garden, on his death the child is in so deep shock that cannot sleep.

Even in older age these instances might occur as with school or college going adolescent who are highly scared of their teachers, even if any mistake occurs then they would be given punishment or mocked at in front of whole class. Similarly, a newly married independent 22nd century girl when goes to traditional, orthodox family cannot tolerate the interference in her life by the members of her joint family and thinks as if she had landed in hell. She cannot say anything to anyone and can neither accept it initially, as time passes she accepts it with beginning of Carcinosin pathology.

They constantly live in fear and develop an attitude not to do anything wrong so are highly meticulous and does all tasks at their best, as time passes it becomes their nature to do every task in refined way (CR – Mentals,

Fastidious) rendering them to become more mentally developed than their age (CR – Mentals, Precocity). They are too nervous and lack confidence feeling that what if something wrong happens and suffers from anxiety neurosis and hyperhydrosis.

The way they dress is impressive, even small girls of 5 years has "Matching sense" she even tells her mother to wear particular outfit and they try to appear at their best with whatever they have. They are not demanding outwardly but internally wish their wish to be fulfilled. A 3 yrs girl came with her mother for consultation when asked what problem brought her to me she told straight away to her mother to go out of the consultation room so that she could talk, in surprise I nictated her mother by blinking to go and sit in waiting room, when I asked her why she told her mother to leave, she confidently told me "Problem is mine and you are to deal with it, what is the work of mother here!" she gave her complete case by herself in first sitting itself, showing her inborn Carcinosin nature.

Instance of fear is also seen in those who were raped (M – Mind, Sexual, Rape, ailments from.) by their neighbours or relative, they have to face them every now and then (M – Mind, Humiliation, (ailments from) rape after.) and cannot say anything to anyone. This constant fear makes one so sensitive that she knows exactly what she wants in life and do not utter even a single word if not given but if her siblings or friends are denied of what they want she takes stand and fight for them, as she is aware of the pain that loss causes. A divorced girl of 30 yrs wished to marry a boy of her dream and her family members were against this marriage, she tried her best to manage everything hoping that everything settles down but failed, although her love was pure for the boy but she could not take stand for herself and suffered from insomnia in which no medicines responded and her health began to deteriorate day by day. After few years, her cousin sister loved a boy and wanted to get married and their family was against this marriage. She took stand firmly against whole family and did all to get them married. Here she revolted against family for her sister but not for her own sake. They are so much sensitive that they can bear everything themselves but cannot let anyone else suffer in same way, they do not revolt for themselves as they do not like to be heard as being selfish and hurt anyone esp. their parents, the one whom they love the most.

We know some broken down families after divorce, the father and mother go their ways and leads life according to their wish but most deprived are their children, they have to sacrifice either love and care of father or mother, those children are like pile of broken glass, somehow managed to be one above the other; a little jerk shatters them. They have so low immunity that they catch cold and infection easily rendering them to suffer from severe allergy in any form, dyspnoea, otitis media, ringworm, urticaria, etc. From early childhood they do not find any vent for their emotions and keep everything to themselves, as they grow up they easily fall in romantic relationship even at times physical relationships to meet their emotional vent and feel that they too are loved ones, and can go to any extent to save their relationship. They try till their last effort but once they fail then they breakdown and some health issues occurs. School going 17 yrs girl came in contact with 35 yrs divorcee boy through social media, they started talking over telephone and had not met him, the girl got so much involved with him that she decided to skip her exams and ran from house, to marry him anyhow. Her father brought her safe somehow from a distance of 100 kms, knowing that he is not suitable for her. When her father talked with her and strictly told her to break the relationship she broke down and landed in PCOD.

Whenever they talk they generally speak "We" instead of "I" – as they relate themselves to others and perceive their feelings so vividly as if they are feeling it. They are even sensitive to cruelty towards animals (CR – Mentals, Love animals, for.). Number of animal rights volunteers are Carcinosin.

Absence of childhood diseases in childhood is important entry point for prescribing Carcinosin. But, after eradication of Small pox came in the concept of prophylaxis and vaccination is forced and tradition of giving vaccination to newborn came into being. We see many childrens do not have their regular childhood diseases like measles or chicken pox, which cannot be taken as indication for Carcinosin unless it occurs to them at older age. A 25 yrs male was apparently healthy in childhood and had chicken pox along with nocturnal enuresis at 25 yrs of age, indicating Carcinosin. Similarly menarchy at 20 yrs or after it, is also seen at times.

Carcinosin individuals who are depressed generally have psychiatric problems in family history. There are some strange points like the person may be highly intelligent or mentally retarded, he may be so neat and tidy or remains dirty. They are extroverted but they can also be introverted if they are having any grief hidden. They may have desire and aversion for the same things, at different times but mostly there is desire for chocolate esp. dark plain dairy milk or dark chocolate, (Dairy milk nuts – Calc phos).

Children are fascinated by ghost and horror stories or television program but the day they see or hear the story the same day on going to sleep they see similar dreams and wake up being frightened in dream relating to ghost. So, this medicine is bipolar and having symptoms too antipodes to each other. This is the core reason of not being able to comprehend it in real sense and take its advantage. Keeping this in mind only those symptoms which I found to be useful in practice are mentioned in this work.

2. CASES, USING CARCINOSIN

a) In Carcinoma cases

Abnormal cells divide rapidly to form changes which are collectively called as Cancer. Cells are abnormally dividing due to any form of stressors acting on them, many times when the stressors are removed or are ineffective the cells come to their normal state and regression of carcinoma occurs. This point of reversibility and irreversibility is unknown as mentioned in texts of Pathology. So any form of cancer can be treated with confidence in Homoeopathy with aim to make the functioning of the cells normal. Numerous cases are dealt with and many gained its normal functioning (Medicines needs to be changed as symptom changes, to take it to recovery.). Here we are showing only use of Carcinosin in cases of Carcinoma so, some cases where it is used exclusively and singly is only mentioned.

52 yrs female complaining of Oedema and thrush for 3 yrs and post nasal drip for 6 – 7 month. She was utterly sleepless for 20 yrs due to continuous fearful thought that something would happen (CR – Sleep, Sleeplessness,

General Thoughts from.). She had B/L rupture of tympanic membrane, rupture initially lt in 1998 and then rt in 2007, then hysterectomy was done due to uterine fibroid in 2007. She suffered from malignant HTn leading to oedema and her weight went up to 115 kgs, presently she is 85 kgs, severe dyspnoea occurred 3 yrs back. She had scorpion bite some 20 yrs back due to which she was unconscious for 12 hrs. She was vaccinated as per schedule of that time. She had lt sided Ca breast which was operated, had completed her course of radio as well as chemotherapy. Her maternal grandmother had Pulmonary Tuberculosis and both father and mother has DM type II and HTn. She was initially chilly but presently hot after chemotherapy, do not like to eat anything (CR – Stomach, Appetite wanting.). If anything happens and she is hurt she cries (CR – Mentals, Weeping easily.) but if anyone tries to make her understand she gets irritated (CR – Mentals, Consolation agg.) and so not show her anger to anyone (CR – Mentals, Ailments from anger, vexation, suppression from.). She was given Carcinosin 1M. After a week she began to sleep. She was kept on Placebo, after next week her post nasal drip was as such but appetite was improving. Again kept on Placebo for a week, now she was having good sleep her irritability reduced and appetite was good but thrush as such with mild changes which goes imperceptible as patient said. She was kept on Placebo and in span of 3 months her thrush went off and all other complaints went off. This case where all treatment was done and still problem persisted was treated with Carcinosin and fetched results.

45 yrs female complaining of abdominal pain for long time. She had been under all sorts of therapeutic treatment without any result. O/P – Nodular growth was felt in her rt lower quadrant. Her USG whole abdomen showed a large well defined multilobulated cyst – solid mass of 110 x 84 mm in rt iliac fossa. MRI showed multiple para aortic peri pancreatic mesenteric and peri portal lymphadenopathy. CA – 125 was 39.2. There was sudden weight loss for 2 – 3 months presently having 42 kgs (CR – Generals, Emaciation, general.). She had ringworm in childhood and tubectomy was done 4 yrs back. Her side is rt, chilly pt, thirsty with desire for chilled water, piquant, salt, warm food and aversion to sweet. She had irregular bowel habits and scanty sweating. Her smelling sense was excellent. Whenever she gets angry she trembles, feels uncomfortable in noisy environment. Believes in God and likes all the things to be done in perfect manner (CR – Mentals. Fastidious.). Her attendant were too much anxious and wanted to go for surgery but the surgeon denied for operation as the value of CA – 125 was more and it leads to chances of metastasis of carcinoma during operative procedure, so they came to reduce the value of CA – 125 if possible. She was constantly crying saying that she do not want to die, her children are too small and she have to live for them. (CR – Mentals, Fear death, of.). She was given Carcinosin in 10M one dose followed by Placebo for a

month. After one month her weight was not decreased, stool became better and pain reduced. Kept on Placebo further for one month, her weight increased to 43 kgs, no pain in abdomen and CA – 125 was 28.8. This reduction of CA – 125 led them to get operated.

While I was studying in Kumaoun University, Nainital, once Prof. (Dr). P. S. Rawat, said that in any case of carcinoma you will find some sort of injury either mental or physical by accident or medications. Since then I look for it in cases and saw it to be true. These at times are intentionally hidden and at times forgotten by patients and his attendants thinking that it would be of no use to physician in his treatment. If these stuffs are known then, the case can be managed well and taken to path of recovery soon.

b) In Acute cases

In laying criteria for acute and chronic diseases in § 72 nowhere any time period is mentioned as we find in works of dominant medical science. Whereas a case to be called as acute shall fulfill following –

- It should have sudden onset.
- It should have rapid progress.
- It shall finish its course in moderate time.
- Either it finishes its course or takes life of the patient labouring under it, due to its violence.

Now, once we know that the case in hand is acute then we see – "most probable exciting cause" which is most important in case of acute diseases as per § 5 and "the straightest way to cure, as certain as that there is but one straight line between two given points." as mentioned in § 53. Combining these two points we come to conclusion that in case of acute disease we need the most probable exciting cause which serves as one point and the other point is the complaint of the patient, now the straight line which will be shortest can be drawn between the two points which comes out to be the medicine which has shown by experience to effect both the cause and the effect at hand. Here are few cases to show the use of Carcinosin basing on above concept in acute.

16 yrs girl complained of acute pain in abdomen for ½ hrs after hearing the news of minor girl being gang raped (CR – Mentals, Ailments from shock.). Attendant confessed that she was molested at the age of 10 yrs (M – Mind, Humiliation ailments from, rape after.). She was very much restless and in agony. She was given Carcinosin 30 one dose, no improvement in 15 min, so again repeated, but after 15 min no change was seen. So, she was given Carcinosin 200, it acted. After 5 min there was reduction in intensity of pain and it was completely relieved in 25 min, without needing any repetition further.

A lady aged 30 yrs complained of severe nausea and vomiting for 20 days after eating and drinking anything. She was apparently fine but the problem started when she saw horror movie with her husband and her husband scared her next night in similar manner as was seen on screen (CR – Mentals, ailments from shock.). She grew very weak and prostrated and felt so scared of vomiting that even the thought of food intensifies her nausea (CR – Mentals, Thinking, ailments, complaints of, agg.). Vomiting gives no relief in nausea and she did not eat nor drink anything. She was given Carcinosin 1M and she reported reduced nausea in 10 min, she got complete relief in 25 min, then she was asked to eat something after an hour, when she felt hungry she took sip of water, there was no vomiting but some nausea persisted. She was kept on Nihilinum and gradually it was also gone. She started to gain weight in a month.

Numerous cases of cyclic vomiting syndrome is cured by Carcinosin with or without supplementation of magnesium depending on its blood value. (A point to note regarding the blood value of Serum Magnesium is that Magnesium is found in RBC so RBC Magnesium value needs to be checked for exact result, but when it is not available Serum magnesium is done and if it is increased in Serum then it implies that it is reduced in RBC thereby if at all Serum Magnesium is normal or increased in Value, it is to be taken as Magnesium deficiency and Magnesium supplementation is needed.)

c) In cases having direct cause effect Relationship corelating to Carcinosin

Cause is immediate antecedent of the effect. By application of Bacon's logic in Homoeopathy we see that therapeutically it works. During drug proving we rarely come across any cause effect phenomenon but on using a particular drug and introspecting its uses we come to conclude that particular cause effect phenomenon is applicable in it. Thereby, this is purely a clinical stuff, coming from experience.

As mentioned in cases of Acute disease, cause for any problem plays an important role in treating through homoeopathy. So if we get any probable cause may be of long time back, but basing on it the medicine when given gives marvelous results. Presenting here such case.

Male child of 6 months was suffering from fluent coryza after being attacked by pneumonia at birth (CR – Generals, Pneumonia, never well since.). He was kept on antibiotics and ultimately the child became very weak and there developed dyspnoea due to congestion of lungs which gradually faded up but the coryza persisted. The child was prematurely born of LSCS and kept in incubator for a week. Child was active and his milestones were earlier in walking and talking (CR – Mentals, Precocity). He was given a dose of Carcinosin 200 followed by Rubrum for 2 weeks. After 2 weeks his parents reported that coryza is much less and he is improving, he was again given Rubrum for 2 weeks. They did not report after that sitting but after a year her mother met in market and told that the boy is having no problem after that dose and is still fine.

d) In Chronic Jumbled up cases where indicated medicine does not act as expected

Chronic diseases have extremely slow and insidious progression which remains throughout the life of patient unless treated properly (§ 72). Patient goes from one physician to other in search for his cure but is left in despair. Physician treating such case, if gets finer points to deal with: then it is excellent; else they deal in Zigzag way. This way of approaching may leads to iatrogenic diseases (§ 74, 75). Such cases where no medicine gives expected results; even though it was well indicated; then comes in Carcinosin as shows in this case.

29 yrs male complained of hardness of hearing with trembling of B/L hands for 5 yrs, he had been under various physicians for his complaints with no results. Ultimately he came under a homoeopathic physician under whom he had been for an year. His prescriptions were not available so no idea of what he had been given. O/E his Plantar reflex, Knee jerk was nil and elbow jerk was brisk. M/E of urine show numerous RBC. He was apparently healthy

since birth, just had ring worm infection in childhood. His siblings have strong history of asthma. He is much thirsty, having desire for spicy items and chocolates esp. Dairy milk. Aversion to sour, his sleep is not refreshing with vivid dreams and lies on abdomen. Smelling sense was reduced and sweating scanty. He does not share his problems easily with anyone and in anger when he controls; he trembles. To start with he was given Blumea odorata Q 10 gtt x TDS for a week to check RBC in urine (Due to anticipation that any untoward reaction might happen if any deep acting medicine is given in this case as I was not aware of the previous medicines given, so started this case with mother tincture.), M/E urine after a week reveal that RBC were nil. He was keep on Placebo for about 6 months then he developed sudden sore throat with much salivation so he was given Merc sol 200 one dose followed by Placebo for 14 days, his sore throat was gone but no change in other complaints. He was on Placebo for 3 more months then he suddenly developed some skin eruptions in which his skin began to peel off when touched, very painful and itchy. He was given Sulphur 1M one dose followed by Placebo, his skin ailment was gone in a week, again he was kept on Placebo with no change in his presenting complaints for 3 more months. Now it had been a year and no change in his complaints, then he was given Carcinosin 1M one dose and Placebo. He was kept on Placebo and in span of 3 months his hearing improved and no trembling in his hands, all his reflexes became normal. It had been 4 yrs, he is apparently alright without any major problems.

This case shows that when a person is with other physician and we do not know what had been given to him then it is wise to start with short acting medicines or any mother tinctures, Bach flower or Biochemics to avoid any reactions. When any specific problem indicates a medicine, then it is to be administered, after the symptoms are gone and patient is not yet cured then Carcinosin was given. Carcinosin when used in such cases either clears the case and provides indication for another medicine or clears the case by removing obstacle.

e) In those cases where well indicated medicine fails due to presence of some obstacle

In treating any disease initially treat indisposition (§ 7), then if disease remains; taking the whole case indicated medicine is to be administered. If indicated medicine fails then obstacles are to be looked for and removed (§ 3). Now, if any case is struck, means there is some obstacle which needs to be taken care of as seen in this case.

An unmarried lady aged 38 yrs complained of numerous vague symptoms for 5 yrs. She had been under various physicians for treatment and they diagnosed her having fluctuating TSH, at times her TSH goes below 0.05 and at times it increases to 15. This huge difference shows turmoil of her mind. Her case was taken and Platina was given basing on her egoistic nature and habit of masturbation, she is not satisfied unless she squirts thrice successively along with other physical generals. It relieved but again there was fluctuation in TSH (Her TSH was checked at every 3 months). Her case was retaken and given Puls. Similarly it acted but again same condition so every time her reports comes and she was given different medicines like Nux vom, Sep, Calc c, Lyco, Staph, Sulph, Tuber bov, and many short acting medicines as per her need, during any acute phase. Still the case is same, some relief but not complete. After 2 yrs she once came and began to cry without saying anything, she cried for almost ½ an hour and then said that at the age of 5 yrs she was raped while she went to birthday party in their neighbour's house. She was shocked and terrified by the pain that she underwent. Whenever she sees the photograph of that day, her parents always tease her that see, she cried a lot that day. Whenever they say such things she feels that they had not taken care of her as they should and never understood her pain rather always made her joke. That day she told her heart out and accepted that the incident occurring at such an age impacted on her largely due to which she could not bear the mere thought of getting married and she think that all men marries to satisfy their bodily desire. So she feels that she is not an article and decided not to marry. Now, her parents were always blaming her for anything that she could not do and pressurize her to take science stream whereas she wished to excel in fashion designing. Presently, she is a qualified pharmacist who did good job in reputed pharmaceutical company at good post in Quality control but ultimately left due to interference of her parents. Today she says that she is of the view that parents shall not just give birth to baby rather they shall be mature enough to perceive the requirement of their child, "Today I feel that I had lost my childhood" she kept on saying and crying, these instance cleared the case and she was given Carcinosin 10M followed by Nihilinum. She was improving after that dose and in span of 2 years her TSH was normalize and all her symptoms went away, even her tendency to masturbation and changebility of symptoms went away. This case shows the importance of obstacle and obvious cause (§ 93) in treating such chronic cases. Now, it had been 6 yrs, she is all fine without any health issues.

f) In cases where constitutional indication of Carcinosin were seen

Whenever numerous symptoms of a proved drug matches with that of the patient's symptoms, as if the medicine comes live in clinic; then it is called constitutional medicine for that patient. Few cases are mentioned here.

5 months old female baby developed vitiligo on back, she loves chocolate (CR – Generals, Food and Drinks, Chocolate desires.) and always wants to go outside of home if anyone goes out infront of her (CR – Mentals, Travel, desire to.). Whenever she urinates or does stool in clothes then she cries a lot unless her clothes are changed (CR – Mentals, Fastidious). She had a greenish brown birth mark on back. She was given a dose of Carcinosin 1M and Placebo. Her mark regained normal colour in 3 months. Now it had been 5 years her milestones are normal and she did not develop any serious disease till now.

2 ½ yrs female baby was suffering from frequent cough, cold and otitis media with fever since birth. She

also had nappy rashes and was vaccinated as per schedule. She was born of LSCS due to non dilatation of cervix and her mother could not breastfeed being epileptic. At 3 weeks of age she was underweight. She had a birth mark Café – du – lait complexion on rt chest below areola. Weight 9 kg. Once unknowingly she took her mother's epileptic medicines. Her paternal grandfather has HTn, and Sleep apnoea, and grandmother has hypothyroidism. Her maternal grandfather had some cardiac problems and grandmother has RA. She is thermally hot, thirstless, she does not eat anything (CR – Stomach, Appetite wanting.), her mother says that she has to run after her to make her take her meal. She desires sweet, sour and plain chocolate (Dairy milk) and aversion to chillies. Her sleep is restless and so light that least sound awakes her, she lies on abdomen and speaks in dream. She sweats from forehead and her smelling sense is acute. She is mentally very sharp and does all works in good pace, likes to go out of house and roam about (CR – Mentals, Travel desire to.). She do not like herself to be dirty, even after sleeping her dress is as it is worn just now, so clean and tidy (CR – Mentals, Fastidious.). O/A – Inspiratory wheeze was heard. She was given Carcinosin 10M followed by Placebo for 2 weeks. After 10 days she suffered from vomiting of food eaten a day before in large quantity. She was kept on Placebo. After a month she had less cold and cough. After 3 months she again suffered from severe otitis media with fever she was kept on Placebo and it faded off in 2 days then came mild cold and cough which also went away. In span of 6 months she was highly relieved and complained nothing, her weight increased to 13 kgs and all was fine. After 2 ½ yrs she suffered from ringworm in rt cheek for which she was given Carcinosin 1M followed by Placebo and it faded away in a fortnight. It has been 2 years she is alright and did not complain of any serious ailment. Many children who are prematurely born suffer from allergic rhinitis and catch cold easily, even at slight change in temperature. They are easily treated by Carcinosin.

9 yrs 8 months old girl was having much lack of confidence and used to be mum in school. She hardly listens to anyone and does everything as she wishes without paying heed to what others say. Her eyes had – 1.25 D in rt eye and – 1.5 D in lt eye, her eyesight became weak after viral fever at the age of one year when she developed cough, followed by dyspnoea and ultimately vision problem. She was only child of the family who took birth by LSCS and was seen to be late in learning to walk. During her gestation period her mother developed weak enamel due to increased fluoride in drinking water. There occurred pustule after piercing of ear. She had dislocation of right elbow recently, and is vaccinated. There is strong maternal family history of hypertension and from paternal side there is strong history of psychiatric diseases. Thermally she is hot patient having desire for chilled water, warm food and sweet. She always takes extra salt in diet, even if all family members think that salt

is perfect but she needs more. Her skin is dry, has white, dry dandruff. Her all discharges were offensive. During consultation she told apparently all the answers without even asking her mother (CR – Mentals, Precocity.). She is good in drawing (CR – Mentals, Artistic aptitude.), does her homework by herself do not miss school and have good handwriting. She is shy and feels uncomfortable whenever any stranger approaches her (CR – Mentals, Timidity.). She loves television program for ghosts and the very night she dreams of ghost and gets frightened and awakes in fright. She was given Carcinosin 10M one dose, followed by Placebo for a month. After a month she boldly speaks in school and now started to listen to others, she was kept on Placebo. Next month her offensiveness of discharges and dandruff were reduced. Now she does not take extra salt. She was improving so was kept on Placebo. In span of 6 months her all problems were gone and weight increased to 30 Kg. Now, it had been 4 years she is doing well and did not suffer from any major illness yet, menarchy at 12 yrs and menses regular.

Male patient aged 27 yrs complaining of no expression on left side of face for 11 yrs with Anti Acetylecholine receptor negative. In his childhood, he had severe attack of fever which use to recur every now and then (CR – Fever, Recurrent history of, Children in). 6 yrs back he had severe head injury and became unconscious. 6 months back he had chicken pox (CR – Generals, Childhood diseases absent or too late) and also suffered from severe ring worm. His father, paternal and maternal grandfather all suffer from Type II DM. Thermally he is hot patient with apparently no thirst. His appetite is good with desire for sweet, warm food and aversion to bitter. His sleep is not refreshing and lies on abdomen, perspiration stains white. He lacks confidence thinking that the other person observes that his left side of face is devoid of any expression and thereby has much anticipation to appear in public. He was prescribed Carcinosin 10M one dose followed by Nihilinum, after two weeks he suffered from fever and he took some antipyretics, fever subsided and his problem became worse. So, he was again given a dose of Carcinosin 10M, this time fever did not recur and he gradually became well, his expression came back and he gained his confidence. It had been 7 yrs that he is fine.

g) In cases where numerous polycrest medicines seems indicated

There are some cases where a number of polycrest seems to be indicated, even repertorization adds to confusion. Selecting the medicine becomes so difficult! In this tough time we see hope in Carcinosin as follows.

4 yrs old baby suffered from dry itching eruptions throughout the body for 2 yrs she had been under various physicians for treatment without any result. Almost her all teeths were effected by cavities (CR- Teeth, Carries, Decayed, hollow, general.). Her birth was in time by LSCS being first baby from LSCS, she did not have mother's milk being scanty and is vaccinated. Her mother has allergic rhinitis, paternal grandfather has Koch, paternal grandmother has HTn and DM type II. Thermally she is hot patient and is thirstless. She does not wish to eat anything and has desire for sweet and raw salt with aversion to chillies and intolerance to any chocolate flavour items; it causes irregular bowel motions. Generally she has scanty urine and sweats mostly from

head rendering the pillow to get wet. She sleeps on abdomen and cannot sleep without holding ears of others. She had great smelling sense. She likes to go out of house and roam about (CR – Mentals, Travel, desire to.) behaves like boys in dressing and walking. She is much obstinate (CR – Mentals, Obstinate, headstrong.) and sharp minded she was already given Phos, Calc, Merc sol by others so this time She was given Carcinosin 1M followed by Rubrum. After 10 days her itching and burning increased and appetite increased so was kept on Rubrum. Within a span of 3 months she was well, there were no eruptions and no scar mark was left behind. It had been 3 yrs, she is all fine.

A girl of 10 yrs came for treatment of warts on right shin bone for 2 yrs. There was itching on the warts and at times it bleed on scratching. She had taken all forms of treatment like Unani, Allopathy, Ayurveda and Homoeopathy without any relief. Her mother suffers from Psoriasis and maternal grandmother had asthma with tuberculosis of intestine and paternal grandfather was having DM type II. Thermally she was Hot patient, who like open air, she feels suffocation in closed space. She has desire for sweet and cold drinks, intolerance to fatty and spicy food causing loose stool. She talks during sleep, frequently changes position in sleep but generally lies on abdomen. She was good in studies and always wanted to be with her mother. She behaves like elder person as if she is much grown up – tells her mother to wear the particular dress while going to party. Even during case taking she told her mother to stop talking irrelevant things and give exact answers. On taking the history she was clearly Puls, her case was taken by some students and they brought out Puls. live from the books and were very happy that they had got the remedy. Others were of the view of Phos and Sulph. On looking the case I too thought that she is Puls, before prescribing I asked her name, while replying she directly looked into my eyes, this instance made me to think that she is not Puls. as a weak, timid, shy Puls. cannot look straight into the eyes of a stranger in this way without blinking knowing that I am physician and all students are standing beside me. Could be Phos or Sulph. She is typically hot pt, so Phos was rejected. Now, she does not have heat of palm and head as Sulph so it was left. On seeing the case again basing on her family history and Precocity I gave Carcinosin 1M, this single dose made the warts to fell in a fortnight, without leaving any scar. It had been 10 yrs, she is fine and did not suffer from any major diseases till now.

3. SERENDIPITY

While using Carcinosin I came across some points which made me to write this book. These I came across by chance. We do not find it easily anywhere. Do consider these also.

I had a chance to treat a child of around 1 month with severe congestion of lungs rendering breathing almost impossible. He was at the verge of dying with fever not responding to any treatment. I told the parents that child may die as it is risky to handle it in OPD but they told that they had been to various hospitals and none wish to admit the child. I asked them to go home and talk among the family members to take a firm decision whether they want me to treat him as there are least chances of survival, they went and returned next day and asked me to treat him without bothering about the results.

He was suffering from breathlessness for 15 days after being attacked by pneumonia at birth (CR – Generals, Pneumonia, never well since.). He was kept on antibiotics and ultimately the child became very weak and there developed dyspnoea due to congestion of lungs. He was a premature birth baby and kept in incubator for a week.

There was cold sweating from forehead. He was listless and did not cry even on giving painful stimulus. O/P – there was dull note on percussion in thoracic cavity and O/A – rales in base and middle B/L lung field.

I gave Carcinosin 1M one dose, with some Placebo and asked them to return after a fortnight. Later on 3rd day her mother came, I was scared and anticipating that the child might be dead, with much internal trembling, anxiety and anticipation I asked her what about your child, she told that he had started to vomit on 2nd day and the vomitus smells of allopathic medicines and syrups, I was greatly relieved by her information and asked her to give the Placebo horis in warm water as per need and come when there is any problem or when the medicine gets over. This vomiting remained for some days and gradually stopped. On 8thday he developed fever and Placebo was continued as before. Time passed and the child had all the milestones in time without any major problem. It had been 10 yrs that the child is apparently fine. This case taught me that Carcinosin acts as a good expectorant where the congestion had taken place, which do not respond to any sort of treatment.

Another case of a 13 yrs child who was diagnosed to be asthamatic developed so much congestion in his chest with dyspnoea that bronchodilators were not responding. He was brought by his mother at advice of another physician. On seeing this child I anticipated that he may die as there was marked central cyanosis and he could hardly breath, I asked her if they had been given any medicines presently, she told that they had been on various forms of medications for about 5 yrs but no results as such and condition deteriorated to this extent. He used to catch cold easily and gradually suffer from congestion of B/L lungs, his expectoration was white and scanty. He had numerous moles in his body. Thermally he was hot and use to drink large amount of water and go for frequent urination (Physiologically if the person is drinking water and his body is not in its need it is excreted out in the form of urine or sweat. In this case the boy drinks large amount of water and goes for urination showing that his body is not in need of water, thereby he is considered thirstless.). He likes chocolates and lies on abdomen during sleep. He is good at drawing and was giving all answers by himself without asking his mother (CR – Mentals, Precocity.) inspite of his deteriorating condition. I told her to take nebulizer if required and gave her Blatta orientalis Q, to be taken if required in 20 gtt along with a dose of Carcinosin 10M and some Placebo. I was much anxious about the child, after a fortnight she came with him, he was looking much improved and had gained weight of a kilograms. On asking about the doses of SOS she told after taking your medicine on reaching home he began to take breath with little ease after vomiting of sputum and gradually he became well, so; SOS was not used. This case too proved above mentioned point.

A girl aged 24 yrs, complained of B/L Hordeolum with severe pain and lacrymation for 2 months, to

Ophthalmologist, She referred her to me as she was having her CS exams nearby. She do not drink much water and had aversion to sweets (CR – Generals, Food and Drinks, Sweet aversion.). Her sleep was not refreshing. She fears of being alone at night and likes travelling (CR – Mentals, Travel desire to).While taking her history it was found that she was engaged 2 months back when she was apparently fine, and when I wished to talk to her regarding marriage she told "Do not tell anything regarding marriage, else it will be running in my mind; I had somehow with much difficulty stabilized my mind in aspect of marriage." Her words made me think that she was not willing to get married but under compulsion from family or some other problem she agreed. Basing on this I prescribed Carcinosin 1M, this single dose, reduced the severity of pain on that very day and in 72 hours it brusted and she was well then. This case shows that Carcinosin is also the medicine in cases of emotional suppression leading to styes. Similar case of a 30 yrs female who was divorced and was on the verge of getting married again with the person whom she loved most; but her family members were against it and denied the proposal. This suppression of her emotions led her to develop severe B/L styes rendering almost her eye lids to droop and close itself. She too got relief by Ign 1M initially but later on recurrence Carcinosin 1M took care of it well.

Carcinosin, has specific action on conjunctiva causing inflammation may it be allergic or due to trauma

(Acon nap., Arg nit.). A male of 9 yrs, complained of B/L conjunctivitis for 5 years when his friend blew red chilly powder into his eye. He took apparently all types of treatment without any results. He was given Carcinosin in 10M and his eyes cleared off in 6 months. Similarly, numerous cases of allergic conjunctivitis cleared up from its use. Another 11 yrs male child complaining of agglutination of rt eye after falling of foreign body followed by conjunctivitis and lacrymation for a year was cured by Carcinosin1M in 3 months.

4. IMPORTANT SYMPTOMS OF CARCINOSIN

History of

- **Premature baby, who are artificially fed and kept in incubators.**
- **Children of broken families who hold their emotions back and are extremely sensitive and defense – less to slightest impression.**

Family History of

- **Very strong history of carcinoma runs in family.**
- **Familial muscular dystrophy, Autoimmune disorders, Psychiatric disorders, Pernicious anaemia. TB, DM.**

Ailments from

- **Victims of rape, sexual abuse, violent punishments, dominated brutally by others.** (Prolonged stress, long continued suppression esp. for infections in childrens, bad effects of mental or emotional shock, fright, reprimands, distressing motherhood.)

- **Iatrogenic effects during intra uterine life.** (Many medicines given to mother during pregnancy, baby live inspite of self medication for abortion.)
- **Grief from death of loved ones.**
- **Violent pneumonia during infancy.**
- **Causeless or acute insomnia.**
- **Headache after child birth.**
- **Chronic epistaxis from emotional disturbances.**
- **From loss of sleep.**
- **CFS, worn out constitution; after severe acute viral infections.**
- **Head injury.**
- **Injudicious vaccination.**
- **Prolonged stimulation of brain causing dullness of mind, brain fag and lack of concentration.**
- **Recurrent fevers which is suppressed for long duration ending with total destruction of immunity.**

Alternating symptoms

- **Alternating sides.**
- **Vomiting alternates with diarrhoea.**

Concomitants

- **Childhood diseases occurring in adolescence or even at older stage.** (Nocturnal enuresis persistant beyond the age of 14 – 15 years or Chicken pox in 25 yrs, etc.)
- **Headache with falling of hairs in young girls.**
- **Teenagers with acne and pimples of face distributed more over the lower part of face and cheeks.**
- **Recurrent apthae in children.**
- **Sleeplessness since first day of birth.**
- **Insomnia with fear of death and depression.**

Mentals

- **Generally reveal history of never being loved or appreciated enough.**
- **Highly responsible and generous having great ability to express their idea.**
- **He is nature lover – very much fond of greenery, animals and breeze; enjoy electrical change, thunderstorm and rain.**

- **Children are easily affected by horrible and sad story. They must be carried or rocked to sleep.**
- Anticipation and anxiety with fear of failure.
- **Precocious; both mentally** (Creative, Artistic, Fastidious, Fear of getting infection.) **and physically.** (Tendency to masturbate in early life. Early development of generative organs.)
- **Sensitive to slightest mental and emotional impression.**
- **Desires travelling.** (Child is ever ready to go out of house with anyone.)
- **Desire to take deep breath.**

Physicals

- **Hot patient thermally.**
- **Thirstlessness.**
- **Generally have desire and aversion for same things, but have marked desire for Chocolate and ice creams.**
- **Aversion to Fruits, Egg, Milk.**
- **Intolerance to Egg, warm food disagrees.**
- Dreams of responsibility as if looking for someone and failing to find him.
- Offensive sweating.
- **Child is generally comfortable lying in knee**

elbow position or on abdomen. (Child sleeps straight on back but in sleep turns to abdomen or in knee elbow position.)

Particulars

- **Soreness in the palate as if a lump.**
- Pain in rectum > pressure.
- Hang nails, nails crippled, distorted, white spot on nails, bitting and pricking of nail.

Observation

- **Adapted to children of dictatorial father or who are deprived of ample quality time by parents for free and healthy personality development.**
- **Useful in long continued suppression of psoric miasm.**
- **Relieves sharp, burning, tearing pains of carcinoma.** (Better in LM – R.P. Patel)
- **Generally comes out as a constitutional remedy in cases of gout.**
- Carcinosin individuals who are depressed generally have psychiatric problems in family history.

On Inspection

- **Café – au – lait complexion** (Generally we see light coffee colour complexion rendering them to look younger than what their age actually is!)

- **Head is broad anteriorly and narrow posteriorly.**
- **Infants with birth moles or bluish spot** (green spot) **with tendency to increase in size as age progresses.**
- **Blue sclera.**
- **Child bites finger nails** – generally he scratches skin near the nail fold and is in habit of abrading it, also habit of thumb sucking is seen beyond the childhood years.

5. RELATIONSHIP OF CARCINOSIN WITH OTHER MEDICINES

In clinical practice Carcinosin comes close to many polycrest but mainly it comes closer to Phos, Tub bov, Lyco, Calc, Sep, etc. Many times person needing Carcinosin is given Phos. as it has much similarities like both the medicine have many symptoms in common but when seen in depth there is difference in apparently same seeming symptoms like –

- Extroverted nature – Carc. is extroverted as he can perceive the need of other person and understand his circumstances, Phos. on other hand is so much energetic that he needs a vent to let it out and wants to embrace whole world so he has an urge to meet new people. So, Carc. reaches out for other's need and benefit and Phos. reaches to satisfy his internal urge.
- Anticipation and anxiety – Carc. has anticipation as he does not what anything to go wrong and listen

anyone blaming him. For him blaming means not loving so he is anxious and has anticipation. Phos. on other had internal restlessness so he becomes anxious and has anticipation by thinking of the thrill that is going to be caused.

- Artistic aptitude – Carc. is inclined for artistic aptitude so that others love and praise him, Phos. is artistic to balance his inner energy and does things to divert his energy.
- Love of animals – Carc. loves animal as they find their best friend in them esp. pet animals like puppy, Phos. loves animal as he identifies himself with them.
- Cannot support injustice – Carc. cannot support injustice on others as they perceive the pain felt by others. Phos. cannot tolerate injustice with them or others as it is a hurdle in their energy pathway.
- Sleep is disturbed, interrupted, restless – Carc. has sleep features as there is much suppressed stuffs within subconscious mind, Phos. has sleep symptoms due to activation of energy of subconscious mind.
- Allergies – Carc. has multiple allergies where as Phos. generally have allergies to strong smell and pollens.

Lycopodium too comes very close to Carcinosin in many symptoms and can be easily differentiated as –

- Have strong sense of responsibility – Carc. has strong sense of responsibility as he longs for love and if he does all task in exact way then all will love and praise him. Lyc. on other hand is known to be person who shuns responsibility but when he knows that if he takes responsibility then he will be getting more and more responsibility, means more and more work, resulting in getting more and more power, then he takes strong responsibilities.
- Offended easily – Carc. are broken down internally due to their hard time in life so they are offended easily, Lyc. takes every offense to their prestige and gets hurt easily.
- Reproaches others – Carc. reproaches others to save herself from any blame and negative situation. Lyc. reproaches others to show his superiority over others.
- Anaemia – Carc. has hereditary anaemia. Lyc. has generally iron deficiency anaemia with assimilatory problems.

There are many symptoms of Carcinosin which is well marked in other medicine, so some important medicines are given to keep in mind whenever we encounter such symptoms with their differentiation wherever applicable.

Victims of rape, sexual abuse, violent punishment, dominated brutally by others.

- Acon nap. – She is frightened by that act and did not come out of it.
- Arn mt. – She becomes stone dead after the act.
- Ign. – She is hurt internally by the act.
- Op. – She becomes life less after the act, on hearing anything or seeing anything.
- Plat. – She becomes more sexually active and gradually becomes sex addict.
- Sep. – She becomes indifferent to everything.
- Staph. – She is much angry by the act and suppress it.

Iatrogenic effects during intra uterine life.

- Acet ac. – Prostration after anaesthesia.
- Nit ac. – Diarrhoea after antibiotics.
- Nux vom. – Irregular bowel habits after antibiotics.
- Puls. – Anaemia after intake of much Iron suppliments.
- Sulph. – Allergic reactions after antibiotics.

Indian medicine in tincture doses Atista indica – When more antibiotics is used and icterus occurs.

CFS, worn out constitution; after severe acute viral infections. Indian mother tinctures like Avena sat – When fever is acute

- Leukas aspera – When anorexia is concomitant.
- Andrographis paniculata – When fever is prolonged.
- Tinospora cordifolia – When fever is repeated.

Head injury. (Head contains numerous neurons so head injury can also be taken as injury to neurons)

- Acon nap. – Impending idea of death after head injury.
- Arn mt – Hormonal imbalance after head injury.
- Calen. – Involuntary retention of urine after head injury.
- Camph – Fainting after head injury.
- Carb v. – Hearing lost, vision lost after head injury.
- Cic vir. – Mind and head symptoms after head injury.
- Cup m. – Brain paralysis with symptom of collapse after head injury.
- Cur. – Paralysis after head injury.
- Dig. – Optical illusions after head injury.
- Hyper.– Neuralgia after head injury.

- Lach. – Giddiness and blindness after head injury.
- Led pal. – Paralysis of iris after head injury.
- Nat sul. – Cephalgia after head injury.
- Nux mosh – Hiccough after head injury.
- Nux vom. – Strabismus after head injury.
- Op. – Apparent death after head injury.
- Seneg. – Effect on lens after head injury.
- Stic pul. – Insomnia after head injury.
- Sulph. – Wretched expression after head injury.
- Tab. – Giddiness after head injury.

Alternating sides

- Lac can. – Symptoms goes from one side to other and again returns back to initial side.
- Vomiting alternates with diarrhoea. Ars alb. – Esp. in cases of food poisoning.

Some important alternating symptoms are found in following medicine –

Asthma alternates with

Diarrhoea, nocturnal => Kali c.

Eruptions => Calad., Rhus tox.

Gout => Lyc., Sulph.

Itching => Calad seng.

Skin ailments => Cro tig, Hep sul, Kal lat, Lach, Mez, Rhus tox, Sulph.

Cephalgia alternates with

Asthma => Angustura vera., Glon.

Colic => Cina., Plumb met.

Cough => Lach., Psor.

Haemorrhoids => Abrot., Aloe soc., Coll can.

Lumbago => Aloes soc.

Menses => Glon., Lach., Zinc met.

Toothache => Psor.

Vision, weakness => Kali bich.

Colic alternates with

Chest pain => Aesculus hipp, Run bul.

Delerium => Pb.

Loquacity => Plumb met.

Rheumatism => Kali bich, Plumb met.

Vertigo => Verat alb.

Conjuctivitis alternates with

Colic => Euph off.

Lymphadenopathy => Paris Quadrifolia.

Rheumatism => Geranium rob.

Oedema => Ars alb.

Convulsion alternates with Rage => Stram.

Cough alternates with

Diarrhoea => Digi.

Haemorrhoids => Euph off.

Sciatica => Staph.

Skin ailments => Croton tig.

Croup in winter alternates with Sciatica in summers => Staph.

Diarrhoea alternates with

Cephalgia => Aloes soc, Podo.

Constipation => Abrotanum, Ant crud,

Rheumatism => Ant cr, Cimi rac, Dulc, Kali bich, Medo.

Skin ailments => Rhus tox.

Dysentery alternates with

Bronchitis => Senega.

Herpes => Rhus tox,.

Memory problem => Phos ac.

Oedema => Apo can, Merc sulph, Medo.

Rheumatism => Ant cr, Cimi rac, Dulc, Kali bich, Medo.

Skin ailments => Croton tig.

Epilepsy alternates with Vomiting => Cituta vir.

Eyesight weak alternates with Deafness => Cicuta.

Haemorrhoids alternates with Heart problem => Coll can, Lycopus vir.

Laryngeal complaints alternates with Uterine complaints => Arg nit.

Mania alternates with

Colic => Plb met.

Menses profuse => Cascara amara., Crot.

Menses problem alternates with

Heart problem => Coll can.

Polyurea => Uran nit.

Mental symptoms alternates with Physical symptoms => Cimi rac, Croc sat., Hyos., Lil tig, Plat met.

Numbness alternates with Pains (Lumbago, Sciatica) => Cham, Graph.

Paralytic symptoms alternates with Spasmodic symptoms => Stram.

Religious affections alternates with Sexual excitement => Lil tig.

Rheumatism alternates with

Angina => Benz ac.

Asthma => Cal seg.

Cephalgia => Ars alb, Lyco cal.

Cold => Kali bi.

Colic => Kali bich, Plb met.

Conjuctivitis => Geranium rob.

Diarrhoea => Rhus tox.

Dysentery => Croton tig.

Gastric symptoms => Kali bi.

Haemetemesis => Led pal.

Haemoptysis => Led pal.

Haemorrhoids => Ant cr, Cimi rac, Dulc, Kali bich, Medo.

Skin ailments => Croton tig, Staph.

Tonsilitis => Benz ac.

Vomitting => Ant cr, Benz ac, Kali bich, Sang can.

Sweat Offensive alternates with urination offensive => Guai.

Generally reveal history of never being loved or appreciated enough.

Mag. c. – Feeling of an orphan.

Puls. – Feels everyone has left him alone.

Highly responsible (Natrum salt) and generous having great ability to express their idea. (Lach., Sulph.)

He is nature lover – very much fond of greenery (Tub bov.), animals (Capc ph.) and breeze; enjoy electrical change, thunderstorm and rain. (Bell per., Lyc., Sep.)

Children are easily affected by horrible and sad story. They must be carried or rocked to sleep. (Bor., Cina.)

Precocious; both mentally (Phos., Puls.) and physically (Hyos., Ori., Plat met.)

Desires travelling.

Lach – Likes to go to cities, malls

Tub bov. – Likes to go to natural places like garden, beach, hill station, etc.)

Loves thunderstorm. (Sep.)

Desire to take deep breath. (Ign – Involuntary sighing.)

Generally have desire and aversion for same things (Arg nit. – Desire and intolerance for same thing.), but have marked desire for Chocolate (Lys.) and ice cream (Phos.).

Aversion to Fruits

Ferr m. – Sour fruit.

Mag c. – Green fruit.

Egg, (Bry – Hard boiled egg.)

Milk (Lac d., Nat c.)

Child is generally comfortable lying in knee elbow position or on abdomen. (Medo.)

By seeing many cases in which Carcinosin is used I found that in numerous cases it acts as short acting medicine and repetition is needed.

Carcinosin acts well after Platina, Pulsatilla, Baryta carb or Baryta Sulph, Lycopodium, Natrum mur.

Many cases requiring Carcinosin are cured but after span of 6 months to 3 yrs there appear some itchy skin eruption or ringworm which is handled by Sulphur indicating that Sulphur is complementary to Carcinosin.

Similarly by using Carcinosin more and more, we will extract its great use in homoeopathic therapeutics and bring out new gems in future.

www.ingramcontent.com/pod-product-compliance
Ingram Content Group UK Ltd.
Pitfield, Milton Keynes, MK11 3LW, UK
UKHW010010090706
13854UKWH00001B/180

9 781639 046287